Fatty Liver Disease Diet Guide

For Beginners

Non-Alcoholic Fatty Liver Disease Preventing, Managing, and Treatment through Diet and Lifestyle Changes.

Title:

Fatty Liver Disease Diet Guide

For Beginners

Subtitle

Non-Alcoholic Fatty Liver Disease Preventing, Managing, and Treatment through Diet and Lifestyle Changes.

Printed in the United States of America.

ISBN: 9798868490941

TABLE OF CONTENT

INTRODUCTION

A condition known as hepatic steatosis, also known as fatty liver disease, is a condition in which fat accumulates in the cells of the liver. The condition known as non-alcoholic fatty liver disease is commonly associated with heavy alcohol consumption; however, it can also afflict those who don't drink alcohol at all (NAFLD).

The most common form of fatty liver disease is referred to as NAFLD, and it has many of the same characteristics as metabolic syndrome. Other components of metabolic syndrome include obesity, high blood pressure, high cholesterol, and insulin resistance. According to some estimates, NAFLD is more widespread than it has ever been, and it affects more than 25 percent of the population of the world.

On the other hand, the consumption of excessive amounts of alcohol is the primary factor in the development of alcoholic fatty liver disease (AFLD), which is the most prevalent form of liver disease in Western nations. AFLD is distinguished by inflammation and damage to the liver, which, if left untreated, can lead to more serious conditions such as cirrhosis and alcoholic hepatitis.

Because fatty liver disease can sometimes lack symptoms in its early stages, some people may not realize they have it until it has progressed to a more serious stage. Fatty liver disease is characterized by several symptoms, including an enlarged liver, feelings of fatigue, and discomfort in the stomach.

Fatty liver disease can, thankfully, be managed, and in some cases even reversed, by making changes to one's diet and lifestyle, as well as, in some instances, taking medication. In this guide, we will discuss the many types of fatty liver disease, as well as their origins, symptoms, causes, diagnoses, treatments, and preventative measures. Alterations to one's diet and way of life, in addition to the use of dietary supplements to promote liver health, will be emphasized here as being very important for both the treatment of fatty liver disease and its prevention.

What Is Fatty Liver Disease

Fatty liver disease is characterized by the accumulation of fat within the cells of the liver, which leads to an overall increase in the volume of fat within the organ. This condition is also known as hepatic steatosis in some circles. The two forms of fatty liver disease that can occur are non-alcoholic fatty liver disease, sometimes known as NAFLD, and alcoholic fatty liver disease (AFLD).

Those who don't use an excessive amount of alcohol are nevertheless at risk for developing non-alcoholic fatty liver disease (NAFLD), which is the most common form of fatty liver disease. Insulin resistance, high blood pressure, and obesity are the three hallmarks of metabolic syndrome, which is strongly linked to this condition. On the other hand, AFLD is a condition that is caused by drinking an excessive amount of alcohol and is characterized by damage to the liver as well as inflammation.

Fatty liver disease can progress into more serious conditions such as non-alcoholic steatohepatitis (NASH), fibrosis, cirrhosis, and even liver cancer. Fatty liver disease is becoming increasingly prevalent around the world, and it is estimated that approximately 25 percent of people around the world have NAFLD.

Types of Fatty Liver Disease

The most common forms of fatty liver disease are non-alcoholic fatty liver disease, also known as NAFLD, and alcoholic fatty liver disease, also known as AFLD (AFLD).

1. **Non-Alcoholic Fatty Liver Disease (NAFLD):** People who do not use an abnormally high amount of alcohol are more likely to suffer from the type of fatty liver disease that is the most common. Obesity, high blood pressure, high cholesterol, insulin resistance, and NAFLD are all closely related to

metabolic syndrome. This syndrome includes all of these conditions. Simple fatty liver, which is usually asymptomatic, can range from non-alcoholic fatty liver disease (NAFLD) to non-alcoholic steatohepatitis (NASH), a more serious form of the disorder that can cause damage to the liver, inflammation in the liver, and scarring in the liver.

2. **Alcoholic fatty liver disease (AFLD):** is the form of liver disease that occurs most frequently in countries of the Western Hemisphere and is brought on by drinking an

excessive amount of alcohol. AFLD can refer to either simple fatty liver, which does not usually cause any symptoms, or alcoholic hepatitis, which is a more severe form of liver inflammation that can lead to liver damage or even liver failure. Both of these conditions are forms of AFLD.

It is essential to keep in mind that persons who consume an excessive amount of alcohol and have metabolic risk factors can have both NAFLD and AFLD at the same time. Drugs, viral hepatitis, rapid weight loss, and genetic illnesses are further potential contributors to the development of fatty liver disease in addition to the aforementioned additional factors.

Causes of Fatty Liver Disease

There are a variety of possible causes of fatty liver disease, and they vary depending on the specific form of the disease.

Obesity, insulin resistance, high blood pressure, and high cholesterol are all signs of metabolic syndrome, which is closely associated with non-alcoholic fatty liver disease (NAFLD). Non-alcoholic fatty liver disease (NAFLD) is also directly related to metabolic syndrome. Other factors that could lead to NAFLD include having a diet that is high in saturated and trans fats, leading a sedentary lifestyle, having type 2 diabetes, losing weight rapidly, and using certain medications. There is some evidence that hereditary factors may play a role in the development of NAFLD.

The most common kind of liver disease in Western nations is called alcoholic fatty liver disease (often abbreviated as AFLD), which is brought on by excessive consumption of alcohol. The symptoms of AFLD can appear after only a few years of excessive drinking. Although the amount of alcohol that may cause AFLD to develop in a person varies from person to person, a higher risk of developing AFLD exists for men and women who consume more than three to four alcoholic beverages daily, and for men and women who consume more than two to three alcoholic beverages daily, respectively.

Other conditions that can lead to fatty liver disease include viral hepatitis, autoimmune liver disease, metabolic problems, rapid weight loss, malnutrition, and genetic diseases such as Wilson's disease and hemochromatosis.

It is essential to have an understanding that the development of fatty liver disease is caused by the intricate interaction of several factors, including hereditary, environmental, and lifestyle factors. The development and progression of fatty liver disease may be brought on by the combination of these factors.

Fatty Liver Disease Symptoms

In most cases, fatty liver disease is asymptomatic, which means that there may not be any obvious indications or symptoms, particularly in the earlier stages of the condition. On the other hand, symptoms could start to appear when the illness progresses further.

Non-Alcoholic Fatty Liver Disease (NAFLD):

A. A bigger liver

B. Tiredness

C. Failure

D. Losing weight

E. Enhanced liver enzyme levels

F. The skin and the eyes turn a yellowish color (jaundice)

G. Spider-like blood arteries that are located within the skin (spider angiomas)

H. Discomfort and ache localized to the abdominal region

Alcoholic Fatty Liver Disease (AFLD):

A. Tiredness

B. Weight loss

C. Abdominal pain and discomfort

D. A larger liver

E. Increased levels of liver enzymes

F. The skin and eyes turn yellow (jaundice)

G. Nausea and vomiting

H. Loss of appetite

You must bear in mind that some of these symptoms can also be present in other liver ailments; hence, you must visit a healthcare professional to acquire an exact diagnosis and the proper treatment. In some people, fatty liver disease can progress into a more dangerous condition known as cirrhosis or even liver cancer. In turn, these disorders might create additional symptoms such as an enlarged abdomen, internal bleeding, disorientation, and hepatic encephalopathy.

DIAGNOSIS AND TREATMENT

Diagnosis of Fatty Liver Disease

It is common practice to diagnose fatty liver disease by doing a liver biopsy, imaging testing, or standard blood tests. A medical specialist may request any one or more of the following tests to diagnose fatty liver disease:

Blood tests: Imaging investigations, regular blood tests, liver biopsies, and other common diagnostic procedures are typically used to diagnose fatty liver disease. In order to diagnose fatty liver disease, a qualified medical expert may suggest the following tests.

Imaging studies: Blood testing: Imaging studies, conventional blood tests, or liver biopsies are the most common diagnostic methods utilized for fatty liver disease. To identify fatty liver disease, a physician might recommend one or more of the following tests.

Liver biopsy: During a liver biopsy, a small piece of liver tissue is taken and examined under a microscope to check for signs of fat buildup and liver disease.

Non-alcoholic Fatty Liver Disease (NAFLD) treatment

The treatment for non-alcoholic fatty liver disease, often known as NAFLD, typically involves making adjustments to one's lifestyle to reduce the accumulation of fat in the liver and improve liver function. Diabetes or high cholesterol levels are two conditions that could be underlying causes of nonalcoholic fatty liver disease (NAFLD), and in some cases, medication may be recommended as a means to address these conditions.

- **Losing weight:** The most effective treatment for nonalcoholic fatty liver disease (NAFLD) is weight loss, which is especially important if the patient is overweight or obese. A weight loss of as little as five to ten percent of total body weight can have a significant positive effect on liver health. A physician may recommend a plan for weight loss that consists of both consistent physical activity and dietary changes that are well-balanced.

- **Healthy diet:** A diet that is high in fruits, vegetables, whole grains, and lean sources of protein, but low in saturated and trans fats, is one way to help reduce the amount of fat stored in the liver and improve liver function. For assistance in formulating an individual meal strategy, a physician can recommend seeking the services of a dietitian.

- **Exercise:** Taking part in regular physical activity can help reduce inflammation, improve insulin resistance, and improve liver function. A medical professional may advise you to seek the assistance of a physical therapist while developing an effective and risk-free exercise routine.

- **Controlling underlying conditions:** Treating the underlying conditions that contribute to NAFLD, such as high cholesterol levels, diabetes, and high blood pressure, can be beneficial. A healthcare expert may recommend medication or other treatments to assist with the management of these symptoms.

- **Alcohol abstinence:** To effectively treat NAFLD, it is essential to abstain from alcohol consumption. Consumption of alcohol, even in moderation, can aggravate non-alcoholic fatty liver disease and cause damage to the liver.

In addition to recommending lifestyle changes, a healthcare professional may also recommend medication that, among other benefits, can improve insulin resistance, diminish inflammation in the liver, or reduce the amount of fat stored in the liver. These medications should not be used in place of making healthy lifestyle choices and should only be consumed following the directions provided by a qualified medical professional.

It is essential to keep in mind that NAFLD can deteriorate and eventually lead to cirrhosis and liver cancer; hence, early detection and treatment are necessary in order to get the best results.

Alcoholic Fatty Liver Disease (AFLD) Treatment

The treatment for alcoholic fatty liver disease is to refrain from drinking alcohol and to make other changes to one's lifestyle that, when combined, have the potential to enhance liver function. Other lifestyle changes include losing weight, exercising more, and quitting smoking (AFLD). The use of medication to treat specific underlying illnesses, such as diabetes or high blood pressure, which are known to contribute to the development of AFLD may also be recommended in certain circumstances. This is because AFLD is known to contribute to the progression of these conditions.

1. **Giving up alcohol:** Stopping drinking is the first and most important step in treating fatty liver disease (AFLD). Even in small amounts, alcohol consumption can aggravate non-alcoholic fatty liver disease and cause damage to the liver. A professional in the field of healthcare may recommend medicine, participation in a support group, or both therapy and medication to help an individual stop drinking.

2. **Healthy Diet:** It is possible to boost liver function by eating a diet that is rich in fruits, vegetables, whole grains, and lean sources of protein. It should have a relatively small amount of saturated and trans fats. For assistance in formulating an individual meal strategy, a physician can recommend seeking the services of a dietitian.

3. **Exercise:** Regular exercise is beneficial for reducing inflammation, improving insulin resistance, and enhancing liver function. A medical professional may advise you to seek

the assistance of a physical therapist while developing an effective and risk-free exercise routine.

4. **Managing underlying issues:** Treatment of the underlying conditions that cause AFLD, such as diabetes or high blood pressure, can be beneficial. A healthcare expert may recommend medication or other treatments to assist with the management of these symptoms.

5. In extreme cases of nonalcoholic fatty liver disease (NAFLD) that have progressed to cirrhosis, a liver transplant may be necessary. A

patient might be taken to a transplant center so that they can be examined by both general practitioners and transplant specialists.

In addition to recommending lifestyle changes, a healthcare professional may also recommend medication that, among other benefits, can improve insulin resistance, diminish inflammation in the liver, or reduce the amount of fat stored in the liver. These medications should not be used as a substitute for giving up alcohol and making other changes to one's lifestyle;

rather, they should be taken only when directed to do so by a qualified medical professional.

Medications for Fatty Liver Disease

There is a wide selection of medications that can be used to treat fatty liver disease; however, the majority of these medications are reserved for the treatment of non-alcoholic fatty liver disease (NAFLD) rather than alcoholic fatty liver disease (ALFD) (AFLD). The treatments for NAFLD concentrate on alleviating a number of the symptoms associated with the disorder, such as insulin resistance, inflammation of the liver, and fibrosis of the liver. It is essential to keep in mind that the usage of these medications should never take the place of making adjustments to one's way of life and should always be done so only under the direction of a qualified medical professional.

The following is a list of typical medications utilized in the treatment of NAFLD:

Pioglitazone: It has been discovered that using this medication can reduce the amount of fibrosis and inflammation in the liver, while also increasing insulin sensitivity. Patients diagnosed with diabetes have typically been instructed to take it.

Antioxidant vitamin E: has been shown to reduce the inflammation that occurs in the liver in persons who suffer from NAFLD.

Ursodeoxycholic acid (UDCA): Research conducted on persons suffering from NAFLD has shown that the supplement UDCA can improve liver function and lessen inflammation in the liver.

Omega-3 fatty acids: It has been demonstrated that people with NAFLD who take omega-3 fatty acids see a reduction in liver fat and an improvement in liver function.

Metformin: Although this medication is most commonly used to treat diabetes, research has shown that it can also help patients who have NAFLD by reducing the amount of fat in the liver.

Because of the possibility that they are not always helpful, the consumption of pharmaceuticals ought to be determined based on the particular requirements and health records of each individual. Patients should discuss their condition with their primary care physician to determine the most appropriate treatment for their condition.

Complications of Fatty Liver Disease

If Fatty Liver Disease is not treated or if it progresses to a more advanced stage, it has the potential to create a variety of problems. The following are some potential problems that may arise:

1. **Fibrosis and cirrhosis:** Fatty liver disease can lead to hepatic fibrosis, which is the buildup of scar tissue in the liver. Liver fibrosis can be fatal. A severe case of fibrosis may lead to cirrhosis, which is a form of liver damage that cannot be reversed. Cirrhosis can lead to a variety of

complications, the most common of which are jaundice, portal hypertension, and ultimately liver failure.

2. **Hepatocellular carcinoma:** Fatty liver disease can on occasion lead to a kind of liver cancer referred to as hepatocellular carcinoma.

3. Cardiovascular sickness can be the root cause of both a heart attack and a stroke, and this condition has been related to an elevated risk of fatty liver disease.

4. **Type 2 diabetes:** Fatty liver disease is directly connected to insulin resistance as well as metabolic syndrome, all of which are risk factors for developing type 2 diabetes.

5. Those who suffer from fatty liver disease are at an increased risk of developing chronic renal disease.

6. Fatty liver disease may make the immune system more vulnerable to infection, which can lead to an increased risk of infection.

7. Increased risk of liver transplantation: In severe cases of

fatty liver disease, a liver transplant, which comes with its own unique set of challenges, may be required.

CHANGES IN DIET AND LIFESTYLE FOR FATTY LIVER DISEASE

To treat fatty liver disease, it is required to make adjustments to both one's food and one's way of life. This is true regardless of the fundamental cause of the problem. These modifications may assist in improving liver function, reducing inflammation, and preventing further damage to the liver.

Importance of Diet in Fatty Liver Disease

When it comes to the treatment of fatty liver disease, diet plays a very significant role. Enhancing liver function and lowering the risk of complications can all be accomplished by eating a diet rich in nutrients, which can also help reduce insulin resistance, weight gain, and inflammation, among other benefits.

The following are examples of the many important roles that nutrition plays in the treatment of fatty liver disease:

- Intake of fat should be limited since eating a diet high in fat can make fatty liver disease worse by encouraging the liver to retain more fat. The function of the liver can be helped along in its improvement by following a diet that is low in saturated and trans fats and high in beneficial fats such as omega-3 fatty acids.

- Increasing the amount of fiber that you consume can help with weight loss as well as reducing inflammation. Fruits, vegetables, and whole grains that are high in fiber can help to improve gut health and reduce the amount of fat that is stored in the liver. Whole grains are particularly beneficial for this purpose.

- Keeping your sugar intake under control A diet that is high in refined carbohydrates and sweets can make fatty liver disease worse by promoting insulin resistance and stimulating the storage of fat in the liver. Keeping your sugar intake under control can help. Bringing your sugar intake down will help with liver function as well as inflammation.

- A healthy weight should be maintained since fatty liver disease is more likely to develop and progress more rapidly in those who are overweight, particularly around the waist. The liver's health can be improved, and the likelihood of experiencing complications can be reduced, by following a diet that is high in nutrients and low in calories.

- Steer clear of alcoholic beverages because alcohol is known to make fatty liver disease worse and to be harmful to the liver. Those who have fatty liver disease should either abstain from drinking entirely or cut back significantly on their alcohol consumption, as directed by their healthcare physician.

Typical Food Recommendations For Fatty Liver Disease

The following is some general advice for those who have fatty liver disease about their diet:

Because it can increase liver damage and speed up the start and progression of fatty liver disease, alcohol consumption should be limited or avoided altogether if at all possible. It is necessary to refrain from alcohol completely or to drink it in moderation as instructed by a medical professional.

Choose the right fats: A diet that is high in healthy fats, such as omega-3 fatty acids, and low in saturated and trans fats can be beneficial to the functioning of the liver. Numerous foods, including olive oil, nuts, seeds, and fatty fish, contain unsaturated fats that are beneficial to one's health.

Increasing the amount of fiber that you consume can help with weight loss as well as reducing inflammation. Fruits, vegetables, and whole grains that are high in fiber can help to improve gut health and reduce the amount of fat that is stored in the liver. Whole grains are particularly beneficial for this purpose.

Foods that are low in fat and high in lean protein, such as chicken, turkey, fish, and lentils, can help one lose weight and improve liver function.

Reduce the amount of sugar and refined carbs that you consume. Fatty liver disease can be made worse by excessive consumption of these foods, which can cause insulin resistance and increase fat storage in the liver. Limit your consumption of sugar and refined carbohydrates. Bringing your sugar intake down will help with liver function as well as inflammation.

Selecting foods with a low glycemic index will assist you in improving your insulin sensitivity and reducing the likelihood that you may experience complications. Foods with a low glycemic index include things like fruits, vegetables, and whole grains.

Maintaining a healthy level of hydration is important because drinking water helps the liver remove toxins from the body, making it healthier overall.

Dietary Guidelines Specific To NAFLD And AFLD

The dietary recommendations and food lists that are connected with non-alcoholic fatty liver disease (NAFLD) and alcoholic fatty liver disease (AFLD) are completely different from one another. The following is a selection of the food lists and recommendations:

1. Dietary recommendations and food lists that are specific to alcoholic fatty liver disease (AFLD) and non-alcoholic fatty liver disease (NAFLD) are related to both of these forms of fatty liver disease. NAFLD stands for

non-alcoholic fatty liver disease, and AFLD stands for alcoholic fatty liver disease. A few of the food lists and recommendations are as follows:

- Fruits include berries, apples, oranges, grapefruit, kiwi, papaya, and pears.

- Vegetables include leafy greens, broccoli, cauliflower, carrots, bell peppers, and asparagus.

- Whole grains include brown rice, quinoa, oats, barley, and whole-grain bread.

- Lean protein sources include chicken, turkey, salmon, tofu, beans, and lentils.

- Healthy fats can be found in avocados, nuts, seeds, olive oil, and fatty fish (like salmon).

2. **Choose foods with a low glycemic index:** The insulin resistance of diabetics can be improved and the risk of complications reduced by eating foods with a low glycemic index, such as whole grains, fruits, and vegetables. The following are some good choices:

- Fruits include berries, cherries, grapefruit, and apples.

- Vegetables include leafy greens, broccoli, cauliflower, carrots, bell peppers, and asparagus.

- Whole grains include brown rice, quinoa, oats, barley, and whole-grain bread.

- Legumes include lentils, chickpeas, and black beans.

3. **Limit or eliminate added sugars:** NAFLD can be made worse by eating and drinking foods and beverages high in sugar because this increases insulin resistance and promotes fat buildup in the liver. Reduce or eliminate your consumption of:

- Sugary drinks include soda, sweetened tea, and sports drinks.

- Ice cream, cakes, cookies, and sweets are examples of desserts.

- Processed foods include breakfast cereals, energy bars, and snack munchies.

4. Saturated and trans fats should be limited or avoided: Foods high in saturated and trans fats can worsen NAFLD by increasing the amount of fat in the liver. Avoid or limit the use of:

- Red meat includes cuts of meat such as beef, lamb, and pork.

- High-fat dairy products include items like cheese, butter, and cream, among others.

- Fried food includes a variety of dishes, such as French fries, fried chicken, and fried fish.

- Examples of snacks that come in a packet include chips, crackers, and popcorn.

- Donuts, croissants, and other pastries are examples of baked goods.

5. **Increase fiber intake:** Inflammation can be reduced and weight reduction can be promoted

with the help of a diet high in fiber. Intestinal health can be improved and the amount of fat that is stored in the liver can be decreased by eating foods that are high in fiber, such as fruits, vegetables, and whole grains. Some excellent options are:

- Fruits include things like berries, apples, oranges, grapefruit, kiwis, papaya, and pears, among other things.

- Asparagus, broccoli, cauliflower, carrots, and bell peppers are all examples of vegetables. Other examples include leafy greens.

- Whole grains can be found in foods such as brown rice, quinoa, oats, barley, and bread made with whole grains.

- The terms "lentils," "chickpeas," and "black beans" all refer to different types of legumes.

Even if it is not the root cause of NAFLD, alcohol consumption can worsen liver damage and contribute to the beginning stages of the disorder as well as its progression. Drinking alcohol in moderation or not at all is best.

6. Dietary Guidelines and Food List for AFLD:

Avoiding alcohol entirely is the most important piece of dietary guidance for people who have AFLD.

Emphasize full, nutritious foods: Inflammation can be reduced and liver function can be improved by eating a diet that is rich in fruits, vegetables, whole grains, lean protein sources, and healthy fats. The following are examples of good choices:

Fruits such as berries, apples, oranges, grapefruit, kiwis, papaya, and others

Fatty Liver Disease Foods to Eat and Avoid

If you suffer from Fatty Liver Disease, the following foods should be included in your diet, while others should be avoided:

Foods to Consume:

Fruits include berries, apples, oranges, grapefruit, kiwi, papaya, and pears.

Vegetables include leafy greens, broccoli, cauliflower, carrots, bell peppers, and asparagus.

Whole grains include brown rice, quinoa, oats, barley, and whole-grain bread.

Lean protein sources include chicken, turkey, salmon, tofu, beans, and lentils.

Healthy fats can be found in avocados, nuts, seeds, olive oil, and fatty fish (like salmon).

Fiber is abundant in fruits, vegetables, and whole grains.

The glycemic index of whole grains, fruits, and vegetables is low.

Coffee: Moderate coffee consumption may help reduce the risk of liver disease and improve liver function.

The following foods should be avoided or limited:

- Soda, sweetened tea, and sports drinks are examples of sugary beverages.

- Desserts include things like cakes, cookies, sweets, and ice cream.

- Processed foods include breakfast cereals, energy bars, and snack munchies.

- Red meat includes beef, lamb, and pork.

- High-fat dairy items include cheese, butter, and cream.

- Fried foods include French fries, fried chicken, and fried fish.

- Packaged snacks include chips, crackers, and popcorn.

- Baked items include donuts, croissants, and pastries.

Depending on the kind of Fatty Liver Disease (NAFLD versus AFLD) and severity of the condition, alcohol use should be avoided or reduced.

It's critical to realize that everyone's nutritional needs and limits are different. It is best to consult with a healthcare specialist or registered dietitian to create a personalized dietary plan that meets individual needs and preferences.

Changes in Lifestyle for Fatty Liver Disease

Alterations in lifestyle, such as those listed below, can also be helpful in the management of fatty liver disease, in addition to food modifications.

1. **Exercise regularly:** Participating in regular physical exercise can assist in the reduction of liver fat, improvement of insulin resistance, and support of weight loss. Aim to complete at least 30 minutes of an activity of moderate intensity on most days of the week. Some examples of such activities include

brisk walking, cycling, and swimming.

2. **Reach and maintain a healthy weight:** The quantity of fat stored in the liver can be reduced, and the function of the liver can be improved, if the person loses weight. Aiming to drop between one and two pounds each week in a manner that is both slow and steady is a good weight loss goal.

3. **Steer clear of or limit alcohol consumption:** People who have NAFLD should abstain from alcohol completely or consume it in

moderation. Patients diagnosed with AFLD are strongly encouraged to give up alcohol altogether.

4. **Stop smoking:** The chances of developing liver disease and causing damage to the liver are both increased when one smokes. Giving up smoking is one of the most effective ways to enhance liver health and reduce the likelihood of developing liver disorders.

5. **Manage other health conditions:** Fatty liver disease is frequently associated with several other conditions, including obesity, high

blood pressure, high cholesterol, and type 2 diabetes. It is possible to enhance liver function and overall health by treating these illnesses, which may involve making adjustments to one's lifestyle, taking medication, or a combination of the two.

6. **Reduce stress:** The development of fatty liver disease as well as its progression has been connected to long-term stress. Meditation, yoga, and other stress-relieving practices including deep breathing exercises and other similar activities can help manage stress.

7. **Get regular check-ups:** The early detection and effective management of problems brought on by fatty liver disease can be aided by routine monitoring of liver function as well as other health markers.

SUPPLEMENTS FOR FATTY LIVER DISEASE

In addition to alterations in diet and medical treatment, the use of supplements may also be an option for managing fatty liver disease. It is essential to see a healthcare provider before beginning to use any supplements, however, because certain supplements may interact negatively with other medications or have unpleasant side effects.

People who suffer from fatty liver disease may find benefit in using the following dietary supplements:

- **Vitamin** E: Vitamin E is an antioxidant that may help persons with NAFLD reduce the amount of liver damage and inflammation they experience. However, taking in excessive levels of vitamin E could potentially be harmful; therefore, it is extremely important to speak with a medical professional about the appropriate dosage.

- **Omega-3 fatty acids:** Omega-3 fatty acids, which are found in fatty fish like salmon and supplements like fish oil, may help reduce liver fat and inflammation in people who have

NAFLD. You can find omega-3 fatty acids in foods like salmon and fish oil.

- Since ancient times, the milk thistle herb has been employed in the treatment of a variety of liver conditions. Milk thistle may help persons with fatty liver disease by lowering inflammation in the liver and enhancing the liver's ability to function, as suggested by a few pieces of study.

- **Probiotics**: It has been demonstrated that taking beneficial bacteria supplements known as probiotics can enhance gut health and reduce inflammation in the liver in those who suffer from NAFLD.

- N-acetylcysteine (NAC): An amino acid known as NAC may help persons whose livers have been damaged by NAFLD to improve their liver function and experience less liver inflammation.

PREVENTION OF FATTY LIVER DISEASE

A healthy lifestyle can often stop or slow the progression of fatty liver disease. The advice that follows will assist you in preventing fatty liver disease:

If you lead a healthy lifestyle, you may be able to avoid developing fatty liver disease altogether or slow its progression. You can reduce your risk of fatty liver disease by following the advice that follows:

- Maintain a healthy weight: People who are overweight or obese are more likely to develop fatty liver disease. A healthy weight can be maintained with a balanced diet and frequent exercise, lowering your risk of developing the condition.

- Consume a well-balanced diet: A diet high in fruits and vegetables, whole grains, lean protein, and low in saturated and trans fats will help you avoid fatty liver disease.

- Limit your alcohol consumption: Excessive alcohol use is a major contributor to AFLD. To prevent the formation of AFLD, alcohol use should be limited or avoided totally.

- Exercise regularly: Regular exercise can help raise insulin sensitivity, reduce liver fat, and promote weight loss.

- Manage other medical conditions: Obesity, hypertension, high cholesterol, and type 2 diabetes are all frequently associated with fatty liver disease. Controlling these problems with dietary modifications, medicine, or both can reduce the risk of developing fatty liver disease.

- Toxins should be avoided: Chemical and pollution exposure can injure the liver and increase the risk of developing fatty liver disease.

- Obtain immunization: Hepatitis A and B immunizations protect the liver and reduce the risk of developing Fatty Liver Disease.

CONCLUSION

A severe condition that can lead to damage to the liver, cirrhosis, and other effects if the sickness is not appropriately treated, fatty liver disease can be a disorder that occurs when the liver becomes overly fat. On the other hand, numerous therapeutic and preventative strategies may be implemented to cut down on the risk of contracting the ailment or to arrest the progression of the illness.

A healthy weight, eating a balanced diet, keeping alcohol use to a minimum, engaging in regular exercise, controlling other health concerns, avoiding exposure to chemicals, and being vaccinated are some of the lifestyle choices that can help prevent fatty liver disease. In addition, it may be helpful in the treatment of the condition to adhere to certain dietary recommendations and take the necessary supplements.

It is necessary to consult with a healthcare professional to obtain an accurate diagnosis, suitable treatment, and efficient management of fatty liver disease. Taking preventative actions can improve an individual's overall health and well-being, as well as their ability to avoid and treat liver disease and manage the condition if they already have it.

Recap Of Fatty Liver Disease And Its Causes, Symptoms, Diagnosis, Treatment, And Prevention

Fatty liver disease is characterized by an accumulation of fat in the liver, which can lead to damage in that organ as well as other complications. The two most common forms of fatty liver disease are known as non-alcoholic fatty liver disease (NAFLD) and alcoholic fatty liver disease (AFLD) (AFLD).

While binge drinking is the cause of alcoholic liver disease (NAFLD), obesity, insulin resistance, metabolic syndrome, and heredity are other factors in the development of NAFLD. Fatty liver disease can cause a variety of symptoms, including fatigue, discomfort in the gastrointestinal tract, and an enlarged liver.

Diagnostic procedures for fatty liver disease typically include blood testing, imaging scans, and liver biopsies. The treatment for NAFLD focuses on weight loss, a nutritious diet, and regular exercise, whereas the treatment for AFLD requires the patient to give up alcohol and make other changes to their lifestyle.

Fatty liver disease can be avoided by making several changes to one's lifestyle, including maintaining a healthy weight, eating a balanced diet, engaging in regular exercise, avoiding exposure to pollutants, and being vaccinated.

Fatty liver disease is a potentially life-threatening disorder that can lead to damage to the liver as well as other complications, but it is manageable provided the correct diagnosis is made, the appropriate medicine is taken, and appropriate lifestyle adjustments are made. By making changes to their lifestyle, individuals can reduce their risk of developing a condition known as fatty liver disease and improve the overall health of their liver.